LOW SODIUM INSTANT POT COOKBOOK

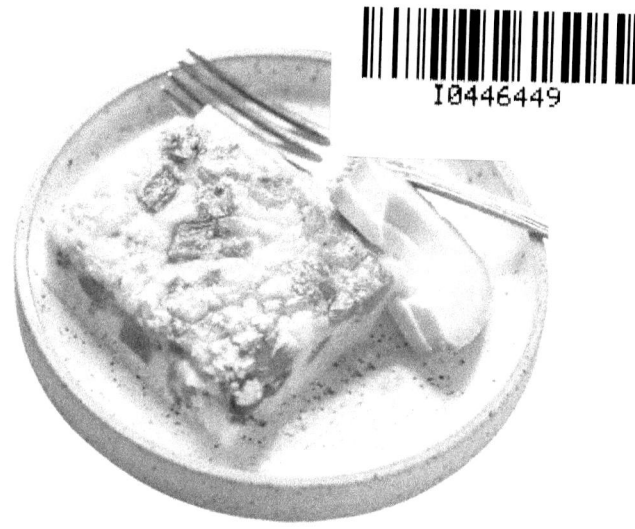

"Mastering the Art of Sodium-Free Cooking with an Instant Pot"

ALLIE NAGEL

Copyright © 2023 by Allie Nagel

DISCLAIMER

This cookbook is intended to provide general information and recipes.

The recipes provided in this cookbook are not intended to replace or be a substitute for medical advice from a physician.

The reader should consult a healthcare professional for any specific medical advice, diagnosis or treatment.

Any specific dietary advice provided in this cookbook is not intended to replace or be a substitute for medical advice from a physician.

The author is not responsible or liable for any adverse effects experienced by readers of this cookbook as a result of following the recipes or dietary advice provided.

The author makes no representations or warranties of any kind (express or implied) as to the accuracy, completeness, reliability or suitability of the recipes provided in this cookbook.

The author disclaims any and all liability for any damages arising out of the use or misuse of the recipes provided in this cookbook. The reader must also take care to ensure that the recipes provided in this cookbook are prepared and cooked safely.

The recipes provided in this cookbook are for informational purposes only and should not be used as a substitute for professional medical advice, diagnosis or treatment.

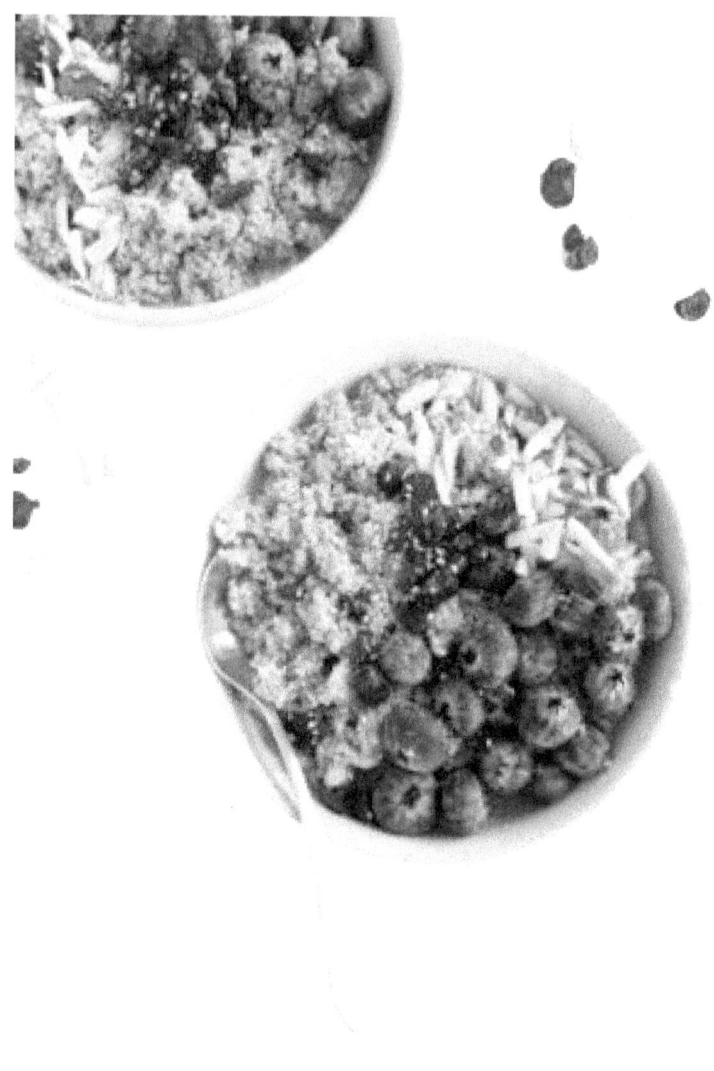

TABLE OF CONTENTS

INTRODUCTION

An excellent way to prepare tasty and healthful meals without sacrificing flavor is to use an Instant Pot with low sodium content.

This adaptable electric pressure cooker, known as the Instant Pot, becomes an invaluable resource for anyone looking to cut back on sodium consumption without sacrificing flavor.

First things first: choosing whole, fresh foods sets the stage for an Instant Pot experience low in sodium. A nutrient-dense meal includes nutritious grains, lean proteins, and fresh veggies.

With the help of herbs, spices, and other low-sodium seasonings, the Instant Pot can turn these items into a delicious meal.

Shorter cooking periods are made possible by the pressure-cooking process, which also helps to retain vital nutrients while preserving the natural flavors of the ingredients.

Adding bold flavors to food while using less salt or no salt at all is one of the Instant Pot's many benefits. Herbs that take center stage, such as garlic, ginger, rosemary, thyme, and others, can improve the flavor profile without using sodium. You may also adjust how much salt is in the dish by using homemade broth or low-sodium broths.

In addition, experimenting with international cuisines that often call for less salt like Mediterranean or Asian-inspired dishes brings diversity and intrigue to the low-sodium menu.

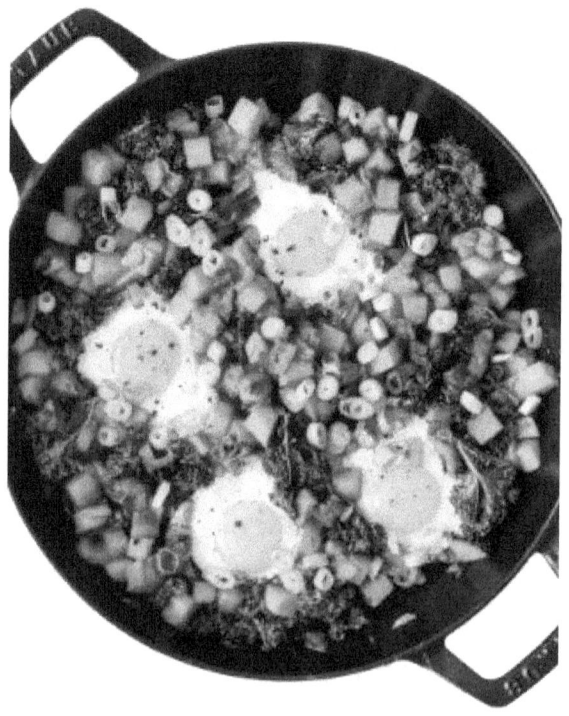

CHAPTER 1

15 THE IMPORTANCE OF LOW SODIUM DIETS IN MANAGING HEALTH CONDITIONS

1. **Blood Pressure Regulation:** A low-sodium diet's beneficial effects on blood pressure are one of the main arguments in favor of it. An excessive amount of sodium can cause fluid retention, which raises blood volume and, in turn, blood pressure. People can help control their hypertension and reduce their risk of cardiovascular disease by consuming less sodium.

2. **Heart Health:** By lessening the load on the cardiovascular system, cutting back on sodium consumption helps to maintain general heart health. Thus, the chance of cardiac conditions like heart attacks and strokes is reduced.

3. **Kidney Function:** People with kidney issues are frequently advised to follow a low-sodium diet. It promotes improved kidney function and slows the

advancement of renal disorders by reducing the strain on the kidneys.

4. **Edema Management:** The buildup of fluid in tissues, or edema, is influenced by sodium, which is important for fluid balance. Edema can be managed and prevented with the help of a low-sodium diet, especially for people who have diseases like liver disease or heart failure.

5. **Lower Risk of Stroke:** Consuming a lot of sodium raises the risk of stroke. A low-sodium diet can help people reduce this risk and improve their cerebrovascular health.

6. **Osteoporosis Prevention:** Consuming too much salt may raise the amount of calcium excreted in the urine, which may aid in the development of osteoporosis. Better bone health is maintained with a low-sodium diet.

7. **Better Arterial Function:** Studies have shown that reducing dietary sodium levels improves arterial function and lowers the incidence of atherosclerosis and other vascular illnesses.

8. **Prevention of Fluid Retention:** The body's tendency to retain water is strongly correlated with sodium. A diet reduced in sodium lowers the incidence of diseases like ascites and pulmonary edema by preventing excessive fluid collection.

9. **Balanced Electrolytes:** An essential electrolyte for nerve and muscle function, muscular contractions, and general cellular health is sodium. A diet low in salt helps to keep this delicate equilibrium intact.

10. **Improved Weight Management:** Water weight increase can result from consuming too much sodium. By encouraging a healthy body composition and lowering water retention, a low-sodium diet can help with weight management.

11. **Better Respiratory Health:** A low-sodium diet can aid in controlling fluid accumulation in the lungs, which will enhance respiratory function for people with diseases like asthma or chronic obstructive pulmonary disease (COPD).

12. **Preventing Gastric Problems:** Consuming excessive amounts of sodium can exacerbate stomach ulcers and other gastric conditions. A diet

reduced in sodium may be beneficial in managing or preventing certain problems.

13. **Optimum Drug Efficiency:** When paired with a low-sodium diet, certain drugs—particularly those for hypertension—may function better. This improves the way that different health issues are managed overall.

14. **Lower Risk of several malignancies:** Research points to a possible connection between high sodium consumption and a higher risk of several malignancies, especially stomach cancer. Eating a low-sodium diet could potentially reduce the likelihood of acquiring these diseases.

15. **Better Long-Term Health:** Eating a low-sodium diet lowers the chance of developing chronic illnesses, improves general wellbeing, and encourages a more active and healthier lifestyle.

TIPS FOR SUBSTITUTING HIGH-SODIUM INGREDIENTS

1. **Use Fresh Herbs and Spices:** Try experimenting with fresh herbs and spices as a flavor enhancer

rather than just salt. Spices like cumin, paprika, and turmeric, as well as herbs like basil, cilantro, and thyme, can give meals more depth and complexity without adding excessive sodium.

2. **Citrus Zest:** To give your meals a flavor boost, add the zest of citrus fruits like lemons, limes, and oranges. Without adding more salt, the zest's natural oils give food a citrus flavor.

3. **Vinegar:** Use different kinds of vinegar, like rice vinegar, apple cider vinegar, or balsamic, to improve the flavor of your food. By adding acidity, vinegar balances flavor and minimizes the need for too much salt.

4. **Homemade Seasoning Blends:** Using a combination of dried herbs, spices, and other flavor enhancers like mustard, garlic, and onion powder, make your own seasoning blends that are low in salt.

5. **Low-Sodium Broths:** When making soups, stews, and sauces, choose low-sodium or sodium-free broths. To manage the sodium content, you can also prepare your own broth with fresh ingredients.

6. **Fresh Garlic and Onions:** To give your meals a flavorful dimension, use fresh garlic and onions. By enhancing the umami flavor, these components might lessen the need for salt.

7. **Lemon or Lime Juice:** Right before serving, squeeze some fresh lemon or lime juice over your food. Its acidity cuts through flavors and adds a tart twist, so less salt is required.

8. **Herb-infused Oils:** To make herb-infused oils, simmer fresh herbs in olive oil, such as thyme or rosemary. To enhance richness without adding too much sodium to prepared foods or salads, drizzle these fragrant oils over them.

9. **Unsalted Nuts and Seeds:** To add crunch and texture to recipes, add unsalted nuts and seeds. They add a naturally occurring nuttiness that enhances many foods without adding excessive amounts of sodium.

10. **Fresh or Dried Fruit:** Using fresh or dried fruit will give your dishes a touch of sweetness and natural sugar. To balance flavors, take into account adding items like sliced apples, cranberries, or raisins.

11. **Yogurt or Greek yogurt:** Use plain yogurt or Greek yogurt in place of sour cream or high-sodium condiments. They have less salt and a tangy flavor and creamy texture.

12. **Low-Sodium Soy Sauce or Tamari:** Use tamari or low-sodium soy sauce in recipes that call for soy sauce. These substitutes offer the same savory and salty flavors without having as much sodium as normal soy sauce.

13. **Herb-infused Vinegars:** To make tasty substitutes for marinades and dressings with a lot of sodium, infuse vinegar with herbs like garlic, thyme, or rosemary.

14. **No-Salt-Added Canned products:** When using components like tomatoes, beans, and vegetables, choose for canned products labeled "low sodium" or "no salt added". You have the ability to regulate how much salt is in your food with these choices.

15. **Try Different Cooking Methods:** To bring out the tastes of the ingredients naturally, try cooking techniques including roasting, grilling, and sautéing.

By using these methods, flavor can be improved without using more sodium.

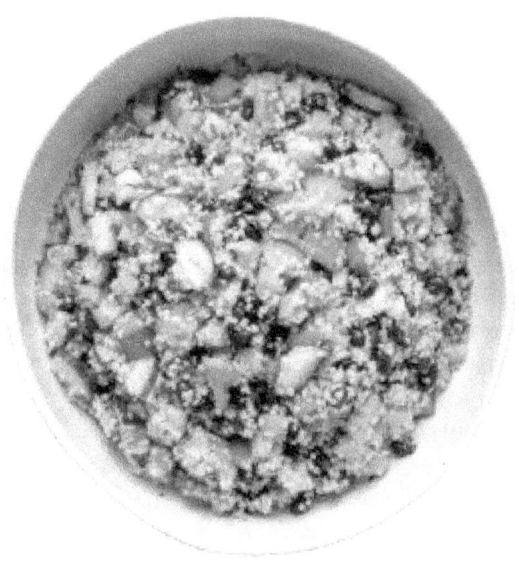

CHAPTER 2

14-DAY MEAL PLAN

DAY 1

Breakfast: Instant Pot Egg Casserole

Lunch: Instant Pot Chicken and Vegetable Soup

Dinner: Instant Pot Salmon with Herbs

DAY 2

Breakfast: Instant Pot Quinoa Breakfast Bowl

Lunch: Instant Pot Lentil Curry

Dinner: Instant Pot Minestrone Soup

DAY 3

Breakfast: Instant Pot Chia Seed Pudding

Lunch: Instant Pot Quinoa Salad with Vegetables

Dinner: Instant Pot Vegetable Risotto

DAY 4

Breakfast: Instant Pot Breakfast Burrito Bowl

Lunch: Instant Pot Turkey Chili

Dinner: Instant Pot Quinoa and Black Bean Bowl

DAY 5

Breakfast: Instant Pot Steel-Cut Oats with Berries

Lunch: Instant Pot Lemon Garlic Chicken

Dinner: Instant Pot Turkey Chili

DAY 6

Breakfast: Instant Pot Sweet Potato Hash

Lunch: Instant Pot Black Bean Soup

Dinner: Instant Pot Shrimp Scampi

DAY 7

Breakfast: Instant Pot Banana Bread Oatmeal

Lunch: Instant Pot Shrimp and Broccoli

Dinner: Instant Pot Beef and Broccoli

DAY 8

Breakfast: Instant Pot Breakfast Rice Pudding

Lunch: Instant Pot Cauliflower Rice Pilaf

Dinner: Instant Pot Lemon Herb Tilapia

DAY 9

Breakfast: Instant Pot Apple Cinnamon Porridge

Lunch: Instant Pot Butternut Squash Soup

Dinner: Instant Pot Chickpea and Spinach Stew

DAY 10

Breakfast: Instant Pot Breakfast Quinoa with Almonds and Berries

Lunch: Instant Pot Chickpea Curry

Dinner: Instant Pot Cauliflower and Chickpea Curry

DAY 11

Breakfast: Instant Pot Egg Casserole

Lunch: Instant Pot Chicken and Vegetable Soup

Dinner: Instant Pot Salmon with Herbs

DAY 12

Breakfast: Instant Pot Quinoa Breakfast Bowl

Lunch: Instant Pot Lentil Curry

Dinner: Instant Pot Minestrone Soup

DAY 13

Breakfast: Instant Pot Chia Seed Pudding

Lunch: Instant Pot Quinoa Salad with Vegetables

Dinner: Instant Pot Vegetable Risotto

DAY 14

Breakfast: Instant Pot Breakfast Burrito Bowl

Lunch: Instant Pot Turkey Chili

Dinner: Instant Pot Quinoa and Black Bean Bowl

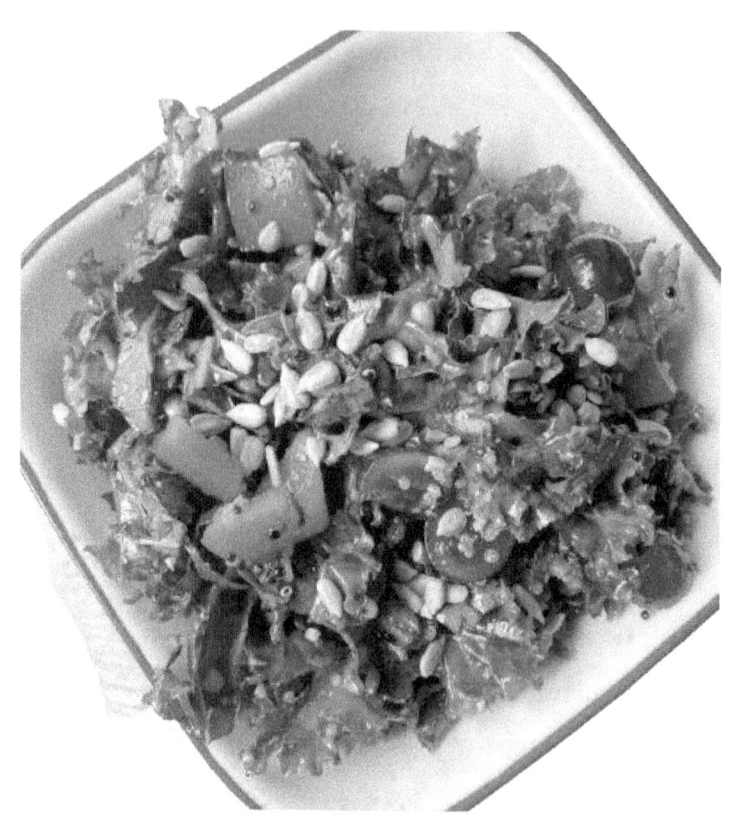

CHAPTER 3

40 NUTRITIOUS LOW SODIUM RECIPES FOR AN INSANT POT COOKING

BREAKFAST

Instant Pot Egg Casserole

Preparation Time: 10 minutes

Serves: 4

Calories: 250

Ingredients:

8 large eggs

1 cup low-fat milk

1 cup diced vegetables (bell peppers, spinach, etc.)

1 cup low-sodium shredded cheese

Pepper

Method of Preparation:

1. Combine milk and eggs and whisk.
2. Include the cheese, veggies and pepper.
3. Add the mixture to the Instant Pot after greasing it.
4. Set the Instant Pot for 15 minutes on manual high pressure.
5. After five minutes of natural release, quickly release.

Instant Pot Quinoa Breakfast Bowl

Preparation Time: 15 minutes

Serves: 3

Calories: 300

Ingredients:

1 cup quinoa

2 cups water

1 cup almond milk

1 cup fresh berries

1/4 cup chopped nuts

Method of Preparation:

1. Rinse quinoa and combine with water in Instant Pot.
2. Cook on manual high pressure for 1 minute, then natural release for 10 minutes.
3. Fluff quinoa, stir in almond milk, and top with berries and nuts.

Instant Pot Chia Seed Pudding

Preparation Time: 5 minutes + chilling time

Serves: 2

Calories: 150

Ingredients:

1/2 cup chia seeds

2 cups unsweetened almond milk

1 teaspoon vanilla extract

1 tablespoon maple syrup

Method of Preparation:

1. Mix chia seeds, almond milk, vanilla, and maple syrup in Instant Pot.

2. Set to manual low pressure for 1 minute, then quick release.

3. Chill in the refrigerator for at least 2 hours or overnight.

Instant Pot Breakfast Burrito Bowl

Preparation Time: 20 minutes

Serves: 4

Calories: 320

Ingredients:

1 cup brown rice

1 can black beans, drained

1 cup diced tomatoes

1 cup corn kernels

1 teaspoon cumin

1/2 teaspoon chili powder

Method of Preparation:

1. Cook rice in Instant Pot with recommended water.

2. Add black beans, tomatoes, corn, cumin, and chili powder.

3. Set to manual high pressure for 5 minutes, then quick release.

Instant Pot Steel-Cut Oats with Berries

Preparation Time: 5 minutes

Serves: 4

Calories: 200

Ingredients:

1 cup steel-cut oats

3 cups water

1 cup mixed berries (strawberries, blueberries, etc.)

1 tablespoon honey

1/2 teaspoon cinnamon

Method of Preparation:

1. Combine steel-cut oats and water in the Instant Pot.

2. Set to manual high pressure for 4 minutes, then natural release for 10 minutes.

3. Stir in berries, honey, and cinnamon before serving.

Instant Pot Sweet Potato Hash

Preparation Time: 15 minutes

Serves: 4

Calories: 180

Ingredients:

2 large sweet potatoes, diced

1 bell pepper, diced

1 onion, diced

1 tablespoon olive oil

1 teaspoon smoked paprika

Pepper

Method of Preparation:

1. Set Instant Pot to sauté mode, add olive oil, and sauté onions and bell pepper.

2. Add sweet potatoes, smoked paprika and pepper; sauté for 5 minutes.

3. Close the lid, set to manual high pressure for 5 minutes, then quick release.

Instant Pot Banana Bread Oatmeal

Preparation Time: 10 minutes

Serves: 3

Calories: 220

Ingredients:

1 cup rolled oats

2 ripe bananas, mashed

2 cups almond milk

1 teaspoon vanilla extract

1/2 teaspoon ground cinnamon

Method of Preparation:

1. Combine rolled oats, mashed bananas, almond milk, vanilla, and cinnamon in Instant Pot.

2. Set to manual high pressure for 3 minutes, then natural release for 5 minutes.

Instant Pot Breakfast Rice Pudding

Preparation Time: 20 minutes

Serves: 4

Calories: 250

Ingredients:

1 cup Arborio rice

2 cups unsweetened coconut milk

1/4 cup raisins

1 tablespoon maple syrup

1/2 teaspoon ground nutmeg

Method of Preparation:

1. Combine Arborio rice, coconut milk, raisins, maple syrup, and nutmeg in Instant Pot.
2. Set to manual high pressure for 8 minutes, then natural release for 10 minutes.

Instant Pot Apple Cinnamon Porridge

Preparation Time: 10 minutes

Serves: 4

Calories: 220

Ingredients:

1 cup steel-cut oats

2 apples, peeled and diced

3 cups water

1 cup unsweetened almond milk

1 teaspoon cinnamon

1 tablespoon honey

Method of Preparation:

1. Combine steel-cut oats, diced apples, water, almond milk, and cinnamon in the Instant Pot.
2. Set to manual high pressure for 4 minutes, then natural release for 10 minutes.

3. Stir in honey before serving.

Instant Pot Breakfast Quinoa with Almonds and Berries

Preparation Time: 15 minutes

Serves: 3

Calories: 260

Ingredients:

1 cup quinoa

2 cups water

1 cup mixed berries (strawberries, blueberries, etc.)

1/4 cup sliced almonds

1 teaspoon vanilla extract

Method of Preparation:

1. Rinse quinoa and combine with water in the Instant Pot.
2. Set to manual high pressure for 1 minute, then natural release for 10 minutes.

3. Fluff quinoa, stir in vanilla, and top with mixed berries and sliced almonds.

LUNCH

Instant Pot Chicken and Vegetable Soup

Preparation Time: 15 minutes

Serves: 6

Calories: 180

Ingredients:

1-pound boneless, skinless chicken breasts, diced

4 cups low-sodium chicken broth

1 cup carrots, sliced

1 cup celery, chopped

1 cup onion, diced

1 cup zucchini, diced

1 teaspoon dried thyme

Pepper

Method of Preparation:

1. Place chicken, broth, carrots, celery, onion, zucchini, thyme and pepper in Instant Pot.
2. Set to manual high pressure for 8 minutes.
3. Allow natural release for 5 minutes, then quick release.

Instant Pot Lentil Curry

Preparation Time: 10 minutes

Serves: 4

Calories: 250

Ingredients:

1 cup dry lentils, rinsed

2 cups vegetable broth

1 can diced tomatoes

1 cup coconut milk

1 onion, chopped

2 cloves garlic, minced

1 tablespoon curry powder

1 teaspoon cumin

Method of Preparation:

1. Combine lentils, broth, tomatoes, coconut milk, onion, garlic, curry powder and cumin in Instant Pot.
2. Set to manual high pressure for 12 minutes.
3. Allow natural release for 10 minutes, then quick release.

Instant Pot Quinoa Salad with Vegetables

Preparation Time: 15 minutes

Serves: 4

Calories: 180

Ingredients:

1 cup quinoa, rinsed

2 cups water

1 cup cherry tomatoes, halved

1 cucumber, diced

1 bell pepper, chopped

1/4 cup red onion, finely chopped

2 tablespoons olive oil

2 tablespoons lemon juice

Method of Preparation:

1. Rinse quinoa and combine with water in Instant Pot.
2. Set to manual high pressure for 1 minute, then natural release for 10 minutes.
3. Mix quinoa with tomatoes, cucumber, bell pepper, red onion, olive oil, and lemon juice.

Instant Pot Turkey Chili

Preparation Time: 20 minutes

Serves: 5

Calories: 280

Ingredients:

1 pound ground turkey

1 can kidney beans, drained

1 can black beans, drained

1 can diced tomatoes

1 cup corn kernels

1 onion, diced

2 cloves garlic, minced

2 tablespoons chili powder

1 teaspoon cumin

Pepper

Method of Preparation:

1. Brown ground turkey in Instant Pot, then add beans, tomatoes, corn, onion, garlic, chili powder, cumin and pepper.
2. Set to manual high pressure for 10 minutes.
3. Allow natural release for 5 minutes, then quick release.

Instant Pot Lemon Garlic Chicken

Preparation Time: 10 minutes

Serves: 4

Calories: 200

Ingredients:

1.5 pounds boneless, skinless chicken breasts

1 cup low-sodium chicken broth

Juice of 2 lemons

3 cloves garlic, minced

1 teaspoon dried thyme

Pepper

Method of Preparation:

1. Season chicken with pepper, and thyme.
2. Place chicken in Instant Pot, add chicken broth, lemon juice, and minced garlic.
3. Set to manual high pressure for 8 minutes.
4. Allow natural release for 5 minutes, then quick release.

Instant Pot Black Bean Soup

Preparation Time: 15 minutes

Serves: 6

Calories: 180

Ingredients:

2 cans black beans, drained and rinsed

4 cups low-sodium vegetable broth

1 onion, chopped

2 carrots, diced

2 celery stalks, chopped

2 cloves garlic, minced

1 teaspoon cumin

1 teaspoon chili powder

Pepper

Method of Preparation:

1. Combine black beans, vegetable broth, onion, carrots, celery, garlic, cumin, chili powder and pepper in Instant Pot.
2. Set to manual high pressure for 10 minutes.
3. Allow natural release for 10 minutes, then quick release.

Instant Pot Shrimp and Broccoli

Preparation Time: 10 minutes

Serves: 4

Calories: 160

Ingredients:

1 pound shrimp, peeled and deveined

4 cups broccoli florets

1/2 cup low-sodium chicken broth

2 tablespoons soy sauce

2 cloves garlic, minced

1 teaspoon ginger, grated

Method of Preparation:

1. Place shrimp and broccoli in Instant Pot.
2. In a bowl, mix chicken broth, soy sauce, garlic, and ginger; pour over shrimp and broccoli.
3. Set to manual high pressure for 3 minutes.
4. Quick release and stir before serving.

Instant Pot Cauliflower Rice Pilaf

Preparation Time: 15 minutes

Serves: 4

Calories: 90

Ingredients:

1 head cauliflower, grated or processed into rice

1 tablespoon olive oil

1/2 cup onion, finely chopped

1/2 cup carrots, diced

1/2 cup peas

2 cloves garlic, minced

1 teaspoon cumin

Pepper

Method of Preparation:

1. Set Instant Pot to sauté mode, add olive oil, onion, and garlic; sauté until softened.
2. Add cauliflower rice, carrots, peas, cumin and pepper; sauté for 5 minutes.
3. Close the lid, set to manual high pressure for 1 minute, then quick release.

Instant Pot Butternut Squash Soup

Preparation Time: 20 minutes

Serves: 6

Calories: 120

Ingredients:

1 medium butternut squash, peeled and diced

1 onion, chopped

2 carrots, diced

2 apples, peeled and chopped

4 cups low-sodium vegetable broth

1 teaspoon cinnamon

1/2 teaspoon nutmeg

Pepper

Method of Preparation:

1. Combine butternut squash, onion, carrots, apples, vegetable broth, cinnamon, nutmeg and pepper in Instant Pot.
2. Set to manual high pressure for 10 minutes.
3. Allow natural release for 10 minutes, then quick release.
4. Blend the soup until smooth using an immersion blender.

Instant Pot Chickpea Curry

Preparation Time: 15 minutes

Serves: 4

Calories: 220

Ingredients:

2 cans chickpeas, drained and rinsed

1 onion, chopped

3 tomatoes, diced

1 cup coconut milk

3 cloves garlic, minced

1 tablespoon ginger, grated

1 tablespoon curry powder

1 teaspoon turmeric

Method of Preparation:

1. Set Instant Pot to sauté mode, add onions, garlic, and ginger; sauté until onions are translucent.
2. Add chickpeas, tomatoes, coconut milk, curry powder and turmeric
3. Stir well.
4. Close the lid, set to manual high pressure for 5 minutes, then quick release.

DINNER

Instant Pot Salmon with Herbs

Preparation Time: 10 minutes

Serves: 4

Calories: 250

Ingredients:

4 salmon fillets

1 lemon, sliced

2 tablespoons fresh dill, chopped

2 tablespoons fresh parsley, chopped

Pepper

1 cup low-sodium vegetable broth

Method of Preparation:

1. Season salmon with pepper.
2. Place salmon in Instant Pot, top with lemon slices, dill, and parsley.

3. Add vegetable broth, close the lid, set to manual high pressure for 3 minutes.

4. Quick release and serve with herbs from the pot.

Instant Pot Minestrone Soup

Preparation Time: 15 minutes

Serves: 6

Calories: 180

Ingredients:

2 carrots, diced

2 celery stalks, chopped

1 onion, chopped

2 zucchinis, diced

1 can kidney beans, drained

1 can diced tomatoes

1 cup green beans, chopped

1 cup whole wheat pasta

4 cups low-sodium vegetable broth

1 teaspoon Italian seasoning

Pepper

Method of Preparation:

1. Set Instant Pot to sauté mode, add carrots, celery, and onion; sauté until softened.
2. Add zucchini, kidney beans, tomatoes, green beans, pasta, vegetable broth, Italian seasoning and pepper.
3. Close the lid, set to manual high pressure for 5 minutes, then quick release.

Instant Pot Vegetable Risotto

Preparation Time: 20 minutes

Serves: 4

Calories: 220

Ingredients:

1 cup Arborio rice

1/2 cup white wine

4 cups low-sodium vegetable broth

1 onion, chopped

1 cup mushrooms, sliced

1 cup asparagus, chopped

1/2 cup peas

2 tablespoons nutritional yeast (optional)

Method of Preparation:

1. Set Instant Pot to sauté mode, add onion, mushrooms, and asparagus; sauté until softened.
2. Add Arborio rice, white wine, vegetable broth, and peas; stir well.
3. Close the lid, set to manual high pressure for 6 minutes, then quick release.
4. Stir in nutritional yeast if desired.

Instant Pot Quinoa and Black Bean Bowl

Preparation Time: 15 minutes

Serves: 3

Calories: 280

Ingredients:

1 cup quinoa, rinsed

2 cups water

1 can black beans, drained

1 cup corn kernels

1 bell pepper, diced

1 avocado, sliced

1 lime, juiced

2 tablespoons cilantro, chopped

Pepper

Method of Preparation:

1. Rinse quinoa and combine with water in Instant Pot.
2. Set to manual high pressure for 1 minute, then natural release for 10 minutes.
3. Fluff quinoa, and mix with black beans, corn, bell pepper, lime juice, cilantro and pepper.
4. Serve topped with avocado slices.

Instant Pot Turkey Chili

Preparation Time: 20 minutes

Serves: 5

Calories: 280

Ingredients:

1 pound ground turkey

1 can kidney beans, drained

1 can black beans, drained

1 can diced tomatoes

1 cup corn kernels

1 onion, diced

2 cloves garlic, minced

2 tablespoons chili powder

1 teaspoon cumin

Pepper

Method of Preparation:

1. Set Instant Pot to sauté mode, brown ground turkey with onion and garlic.

2. Add kidney beans, black beans, tomatoes, corn, chili powder, cumin and pepper; stir well.

3. Close the lid, set to manual high pressure for 10 minutes, then quick release.

Instant Pot Shrimp Scampi

Preparation Time: 15 minutes

Serves: 4

Calories: 210

Ingredients:

1 pound shrimp, peeled and deveined

4 tablespoons unsalted butter

4 cloves garlic, minced

1/2 cup chicken broth (low-sodium)

Juice of 2 lemons

1/4 cup fresh parsley, chopped

Pepper

Method of Preparation:

1. Set Instant Pot to sauté mode, melt butter, and sauté garlic until fragrant.
2. Add shrimp, chicken broth, lemon juice SSand pepper.
3. Stir well.
4. Close the lid, set to manual high pressure for 1 minute, then quick release.
5. Stir in fresh parsley before serving.

Instant Pot Beef and Broccoli

Preparation Time: 25 minutes

Serves: 4

Calories: 320

Ingredients:

1 pound beef sirloin, thinly sliced

1/2 cup low-sodium soy sauce

1/4 cup hoisin sauce

2 tablespoons honey

3 cloves garlic, minced

1 teaspoon ginger, grated

1 cup beef broth (low-sodium)

2 cups broccoli florets

2 tablespoons cornstarch

Method of Preparation:

1. In a bowl, mix soy sauce, hoisin sauce, honey, garlic, ginger, and beef broth.
2. Place beef in Instant Pot, pour sauce over it, and add broccoli.
3. Close the lid, set to manual high pressure for 8 minutes, then quick release.
4. Mix cornstarch with a bit of water and stir into the pot to thicken the sauce.

Instant Pot Lemon Herb Tilapia

Preparation Time: 10 minutes

Serves: 4

Calories: 150

Ingredients:

4 tilapia fillets

1 lemon, sliced

2 tablespoons olive oil

2 cloves garlic, minced

1 teaspoon dried thyme

1 teaspoon dried rosemary

Pepper

Method of Preparation:

1. Season tilapia fillets with pepper, thyme, and rosemary.
2. Drizzle olive oil in the Instant Pot, place tilapia fillets, and top with lemon slices.
3. Close the lid, set to manual high pressure for 3 minutes.
4. Quick release and serve with herbs from the pot.

Instant Pot Chickpea and Spinach Stew

Preparation Time: 15 minutes

Serves: 6

Calories: 180

Ingredients:

2 cans chickpeas, drained and rinsed

1 onion, chopped

2 cloves garlic, minced

1 can diced tomatoes

4 cups low-sodium vegetable broth

1 teaspoon cumin

1 teaspoon paprika

4 cups fresh spinach

Pepper

Method of Preparation:

1. Set Instant Pot to sauté mode, add onion and garlic; sauté until softened.
2. Add chickpeas, diced tomatoes, vegetable broth, cumin, paprika and pepper; stir well.
3. Close the lid, set to manual high pressure for 5 minutes, then quick release.
4. Stir in fresh spinach until wilted before serving.

Instant Pot Cauliflower and Chickpea Curry

Preparation Time: 20 minutes

Serves: 4

Calories: 220

Ingredients:

1 head cauliflower, cut into florets

1 can chickpeas, drained and rinsed

1 onion, chopped

2 cloves garlic, minced

1 can diced tomatoes

1 can coconut milk

2 tablespoons curry powder

1 teaspoon turmeric

Pepper

Method of Preparation:

1. Set Instant Pot to sauté mode, add onion and garlic; sauté until softened.
2. Add cauliflower, chickpeas, diced tomatoes, coconut milk, curry powder, turmeric, salt, and pepper; stir well.
3. Close the lid, set to manual high pressure for 6 minutes, then quick release.

DESSERTS

Instant Pot Rice Pudding

Preparation Time: 10 minutes

Serves: 6

Calories: 200

Ingredients:

1 cup white rice

4 cups low-fat milk

1/2 cup sugar

1 teaspoon vanilla extract

1/2 teaspoon cinnamon

1/4 teaspoon nutmeg

Method of Preparation:

1. Rinse rice under cold water.
2. Combine rice, milk, sugar, vanilla extract, cinnamon and nutmeg in the Instant Pot.
3. Close the lid, set to manual high pressure for 12 minutes.
4. Allow natural release for 10 minutes, then quick release.
5. Stir the pudding and let it cool before serving.

Low-Sodium Instant Pot Cheesecake

Preparation Time: 20 minutes

Serves: 8

Calories: 250

Ingredients:

2 cups low-fat cream cheese, softened

1/2 cup sugar

2 tablespoons all-purpose flour

2 eggs

1 teaspoon vanilla extract

1 cup low-fat sour cream

1 tablespoon lemon juice

Method of Preparation:

1. In a bowl, beat cream cheese, sugar, and flour until smooth.

2. Add eggs one at a time, then mix in vanilla extract, sour cream, and lemon juice.

3. Grease a springform pan and pour in the mixture.

4. Add 1 cup of water to the Instant Pot, place the trivet, and put the cheesecake on top.

5. Close the lid, set to manual high pressure for 30 minutes, then natural release for 10 minutes.

6. Refrigerate the cheesecake for at least 4 hours before serving.

Instant Pot Poached Pears

Preparation Time: 15 minutes

Serves: 4

Calories: 120

Ingredients:

4 ripe but firm pears, peeled and halved

1 cup red wine

1/2 cup water

1/4 cup honey

1 cinnamon stick

2 cloves

1 teaspoon vanilla extract

Method of Preparation:

1. In the Instant Pot, combine red wine, water, honey, cinnamon stick, cloves, and vanilla extract.
2. Add the pear halves, ensuring they are well coated.
3. Close the lid, set to manual high pressure for 5 minutes, then quick release.
4. Carefully remove the pears and simmer the liquid until it thickens into a syrup.
5. Serve the pears drizzled with the syrup.

Instant Pot Berry Compote

Preparation Time: 5 minutes

Serves: 4

Calories: 50

Ingredients:

2 cups mixed berries (strawberries, blueberries, raspberries)

1/4 cup honey

1 tablespoon lemon juice

1 teaspoon vanilla extract

Method of Preparation:

1. In the Instant Pot, combine mixed berries, honey, lemon juice, and vanilla extract.
2. Close the lid, set to manual high pressure for 2 minutes, then quick release.
3. Mash the berries gently with a fork to reach your desired consistency.
4. Allow the compote to cool before serving.

Instant Pot Pumpkin Custard

Preparation Time: 10 minutes

Serves: 6

Calories: 130

Ingredients:

1 can (15 oz) pumpkin puree

2/3 cup low-fat milk

1/2 cup maple syrup

2 eggs

1 teaspoon vanilla extract

1 teaspoon cinnamon

1/2 teaspoon nutmeg

Method of Preparation:

1. In a bowl, whisk together pumpkin puree, milk, maple syrup, eggs, vanilla extract, cinnamon and nutmeg.
2. Pour the mixture into ramekins or a baking dish that fits inside the Instant Pot.
3. Add 1 cup of water to the Instant Pot, place the trivet, and put the custard container on top.
4. Close the lid, set to manual high pressure for 12 minutes, then natural release for 5 minutes.
5. Refrigerate the custard for at least 2 hours before serving.

SOUPS AND STEWS

Split Pea Soup

Preparation Time: 15 minutes

Serves: 6

Calories: 220

Ingredients:

1-pound dried split peas, rinsed

1 ham hock or smoked turkey leg

1 onion, chopped

2 carrots, diced

2 celery stalks, chopped

2 cloves garlic, minced

8 cups low-sodium vegetable broth

1 teaspoon thyme

Pepper

Method of Preparation:

1. Combine split peas, ham hock or turkey leg, onion, carrots, celery, garlic, vegetable broth, thyme and pepper in the Instant Pot.
2. Close the lid, set to manual high pressure for 15 minutes.
3. Allow natural release for 10 minutes, then quick release.
4. Remove ham hock or turkey leg, shred the meat, and return it to the soup before serving.

Butternut Squash Soup

Preparation Time: 20 minutes

Serves: 6

Calories: 150

Ingredients:

1 medium butternut squash, peeled and diced

1 onion, chopped

2 carrots, diced

2 apples, peeled and chopped

4 cups low-sodium vegetable broth

1 teaspoon cinnamon

1/2 teaspoon nutmeg

Pepper

Method of Preparation:

1. Combine butternut squash, onion, carrots, apples, vegetable broth, cinnamon, nutmeg, salt, and pepper in the Instant Pot.
2. Set to manual high pressure for 10 minutes.
3. Allow natural release for 10 minutes, then quick release.
4. Blend the soup until smooth using an immersion blender before serving.

Black Bean Soup

Preparation Time: 15 minutes

Serves: 5

Calories: 180

Ingredients:

2 cans black beans, drained and rinsed

1 onion, chopped

2 carrots, diced

2 celery stalks, chopped

2 cloves garlic, minced

4 cups low-sodium vegetable broth

1 teaspoon cumin

1 teaspoon chili powder

Pepper

Method of Preparation:

1. Set Instant Pot to sauté mode, add onion, celery, and garlic; sauté until softened.
2. Add black beans, carrots, vegetable broth, cumin, chili powder and pepper.
3. Stir well.
4. Close the lid, set to manual high pressure for 8 minutes, then quick release.

5. Blend a portion of the soup using an immersion blender for a thicker consistency before serving.

Potato Leek Soup

Preparation Time: 15 minutes

Serves: 6

Calories: 180

Ingredients:

4 leeks, cleaned and sliced

4 potatoes, peeled and diced

1 onion, chopped

2 cloves garlic, minced

4 cups low-sodium vegetable broth

1 teaspoon thyme

Pepper

1 cup low-fat milk (optional)

Method of Preparation:

1. Set Instant Pot to sauté mode, add leeks, onion, and garlic; sauté until softened.
2. Add potatoes, vegetable broth, thyme and pepper; stir well.
3. Close the lid, set to manual high pressure for 8 minutes.
4. Allow natural release for 5 minutes, then quick release.
5. Use an immersion blender to puree the soup until smooth. Stir in milk if desired before serving.

Moroccan Chickpea Stew

Preparation Time: 20 minutes

Serves: 5

Calories: 220

Ingredients:

2 cans chickpeas, drained and rinsed

1 onion, chopped

2 carrots, diced

2 cloves garlic, minced

1 can diced tomatoes

1 cup butternut squash, diced

4 cups low-sodium vegetable broth

1 teaspoon cumin

1 teaspoon coriander

1/2 teaspoon cinnamon

Pepper

Method of Preparation:

1. Set Instant Pot to sauté mode, add onion and garlic; sauté until softened.
2. Add chickpeas, carrots, tomatoes, butternut squash, vegetable broth, cumin, coriander, cinnamon and pepper; stir well.
3. Close the lid, set to manual high pressure for 10 minutes, then quick release.
4. If necessary, adjust seasoning, before serving.

CONCLUSION

Finally, if you're looking to lead a heart-healthy lifestyle, starting a low-sodium cooking journey with the Instant Pot has not only completely changed the way you cook, but it has also unlocked a world of delicious possibilities.

This cookbook is proof that flavor and inventiveness in cooking don't have to be sacrificed in the name of cutting sodium.

Through utilizing the capabilities of the Instant Pot, I've found a variety of creative ways to add taste to food without sacrificing health.

I've had the opportunity to delve into the art of seasoning with herbs, spices, and other healthful ingredients to enhance the flavor of every meal in this book.

You may now more easily than ever adopt a thoughtful and heart-conscious attitude to your nutritional choices through the quickness and simplicity of the instant pot.

Ultimately, let this book to be your guide while you travel the route of a lower sodium intake. I hope it gives you more self-assurance in the kitchen and encourages you to experiment with your favorite dishes, modifying them to fit your health objectives.